YOUR KNOWLEDGE HAS VALUE

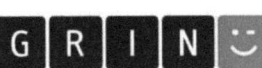

Ocular Drug Delivery Systems

Manish Kumar

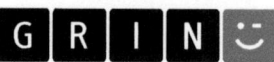

Bibliographic information published by the German National Library:

The German National Library lists this publication in the National Bibliography; detailed bibliographic data are available on the Internet at http://dnb.dnb.de.

ISBN: 9783346902733
This book is also available as an ebook.

© GRIN Publishing GmbH
Trappentreustraße 1
80339 München

Print and binding: Books on Demand GmbH, Norderstedt, Germany
Printed on acid-free paper from responsible sources.

The present work has been carefully prepared. Nevertheless, authors and publishers do not incur liability for the correctness of information, notes, links and advice as well as any printing errors.

GRIN web shop: https://www.grin.com/document/1369759

OCULAR DRUG DELIVERY SYSTEMS

NEED FOR OCULAR DRUG DELIVERY SYSTEMS

Amongst the various routes of drug delivery, the field of ophthalmic drug delivery is one of the most interesting and challenging endeavors found by the pharmaceutical formulator due to unusual pharmacodynamic as well as pharmacokinetic properties and critical environment that exist in the eye (Meqi et al., 2002). Drug administration to ophthalmic region is mainly interfered by its anatomical and physiological features (Nanjawade et al., 2007). For centuries most ocular treatments consisted of ophthalmic solution, suspension, and semisolid for the topical administration of active drugs to the tissues around the ocular cavity. The practical reasons for selecting solutions are the favorable cost advantage, the greater simplicity of formulation production and the good acceptance by patients despite a little blurring (Fitzgerald et al., 1994). As these dosage forms are easy to instill but suffer from the inherent drawback that the majority of the medication they contain is immediately diluted in the tear film and thus rapidly drained away from the precorneal cavity by constant tear flow and lacrimo-nasal drainage.

Therefore, the target tissue absorbs a very small fraction of instilled dose. Due to this reason, concentrated solutions and frequent dosing are required to obtain adequate level of therapeutic effect (Chein et al, 1992).

1.2 ANATOMICAL AND PHYSIOLOGICAL CONSTRAINTS TO TOPICAL OCULAR DRUG THERAPY

1.2.1 The Anatomy of the Eye (Tortora et al., 2003, Wagh et al., 2001)

The eyeball measures about 2.5 cm in diameter, only a small portion (about 1/6[th]part) of the globular eye is exposed in front, the rest is hidden in bony

1

socket of the orbit on a cushion of fat and connective tissue. The wall of the human eyeball consists essentially of three layers: Fibrous tunic, Vascular tunic and Retina (Figure 1.1).

This image has been removed due to copyright issues.

Figure 1.1 Structure of Eye-Ball

1.2.1.1 Fibrous Tunic

Fibrous tunic, the outermost coat of the eyeball, consists of the anterior cornea and posterior sclera. The cornea is a transparent coat that covers the colored iris. Cornea mainly consists of the following structures from the front to back, (I) Epithelium, (II)Bowman's membrane, (III) Stroma, (IV) Descemet's Membrane, (V)Endothelium. The cornea is 0.5 to 1mm in thickness and normally it possesses no blood vessels except at the cornea sclera junction. The sclera, the "white" of the eye, is a layer of dense connective tissue made up densely of collagen fibers and fibroblasts. The sclera covers the entire eyeball except the cornea. At the junction of the sclera and cornea is an opening known as the sclera venous sinus (canal of Schelmm).

1.2.1.2 Vascular Tunic

This middle layer is mainly vascular, consisting of the choroid, ciliary body and iris. Choroid lines the posterior five-sixths of the inner surface of the sclera. It is very rich in blood vessels.

Ciliary body is the anterior continuation of the choroids consisting of ciliary muscle and secretary epithelial cells. The major function of the ciliary body is the production of aqueous humor. Systemic drugs enter the anterior and

2

posterior chambers largely by passing through the ciliary body vasculature and then diffusing in to the iris where they can enter the aqueous humor. The ciliary body is one of the major ocular ounces of drug-metabolizing enzymes, responsible for drug detoxification and removal from the eye.

Iris is the visible colored part of the eye and extends interiorly from the ciliary body lying behind the cornea and in front of the lens. The pigment granules of the iris epithelium absorb light as well as lipophilic drugs. This type of binding is characteristically reversible, allowing release of drug overtime. As a result, the iris can serve as a reservoir for some drugs, concentrating and then releasing them for longer than otherwise expected.

The innermost layer is the retina, consisting of the essential nervous system responsible for vision. Retina lines the posterior three quarters of the eyeball and are the beginning of the visual pathway.

1.2.1.3 Retina
The retina is situated between the clear vitreous humor in its inner surface and the choroids on its outer surface. Retina consists of two distinct chambers, anterior and posterior (Fulcher et al., 2003). Behind the pupil and iris, within the cavity of the eyeball, is the lens. Protein called crystalline, arranged like the layers of an onion, make up the lens. The lens is held in place by the zonules, which run from the ciliary body and fuse into the outer layer of the lens capsule. The lens tends to develop cataract or opacities with age, interfering with vision.

1.2.2 Interior of The Eyeball
The lens divides the interior of the eyeball into two cavities; Anterior cavity and Vitrous chamber.

The anterior cavity consists of two chambers, the anterior chamber that lies between the cornea and the iris. The posterior chamber that lies behind the iris and in front of the lens. Aqueous humor is formed by ciliary bodies and occupies the posterior and anterior chambers, having a volume of about 0.2mL. The fluid is constantly generated by pigmented and non- pigmented epithelium of ciliary body.

The Vitreous chamber is filled with a viscous fluid, vitreous humor, which is a viscoelastic connective tissue composed of small amounts of glycosamino glycans, including of hyaluronic acid and proteins such as collagen (Fulcher et al., 2003).

The conjunctiva membrane covers the outer surface of the white portion of the eye and the inner surface of the eyelids. In most places it is loosely attached and thereby permits free movement of the eyeball, this makes possible sub conjunctival injection. The conjunctiva forms an inferior and a superior sac except for the cornea, the conjunctiva is the most exposed portion of the eye.

1.2.4 Aqueous Humor

The aqueous humor is a jelly-like substance located in the outer/front chamber of the eye. It is a watery fluid that fills the "anterior chamber of the eye" which is located immediately behind the cornea and in front of the lens. The aqueous humor is very slightly alkaline salt solution that includes tiny quantities of sodium and chloride ions. In human eye, the rate of aqueous humor turnover is approximately 1 – 1.5% of the anterior chamber volume per minute.

1.3 ABSORPTION OF DRUGS IN EYE

It is often assumed that drugs administered into the eye are rapidly and totally absorbed. However, contrary to this belief, the moment drug is placed in lower cul-de-sac of eye, several factors immediately begins to affect the bioavailability of drug. Absorption of drugs takes place either through corneal or non-corneal routes. The non-corneal route involves absorption across the sclera and conjunctiva into the intraocular tissues. This route is however, not productive as it restrains the entry of drug into aqueous humor. Maximum absorption thus takes place through cornea, which leads the drug into aqueous humor. The goal of ophthalmic drug delivery system has traditionally been to maximize ocular drug absorption rather than to minimize the systemic absorption.

1.4 DRUG ELIMINATION FROM LACRIMAL FLUID

Ophthalmic liquid dosage forms like solutions, suspensions or liposomes are either drained from conjunctival sac into nasolacrimal duct or are cleared from precorneal area resulting in poor bioavailability of drugs. Drugs are mainly eliminated from the precorneal lacrimal fluid by solution drainage, lacrimation and non-productive absorption to the conjunctiva of the eye. These factors and the corneal barrier limit the penetration of the topically administered drug into the eye. Only a few percentage of applied dose is delivered into intraocular tissue, while the major part (50-100%) of the dose is absorbed in systemic route. Precorneal constraints include:

- Spillage of drug by overflow.
- Dilution of drug by tear turnover.
- Nasolacrimal drainage / systemic drug absorption.
- Conjunctival absorption.
- Enzymatic metabolism.

1.4.1 Transcorneal Penetration

Transcorneal penetration of drug is mainly affected by corneal barriers, physiochemical properties of drugs and active ion transport systems present at cornea.

1.4.1.1 Corneal Barriers

Corneal epithelium is the main barrier for drug absorption into eye. Corneal epithelium acts as a protective barrier against foreign molecules and also as a barrier to ion transport. The corneal epithelium consists of a basal layer of columnar cells, squamous cells, and polygonal shaped superficial cells.

In a healthy corneal epithelium, intracellular tight junctions completely surrounds the most superficial cells, nevertheless the intracellular spaces are wider between wing cells and basal cells. These allow the paracellular diffusion of large molecules through these layers of cell only. Tight junctions serve as a selective barrier for small molecules and they completely prevent the diffusion of macro molecules via the paracellular route. Corneal stroma is a highly hydrophilic tissue; it acts as a rate limiting barrier for ocular absorption of most lipophilic drugs. The corneal endothelium is responsible for maintaining normal corneal hydration (Figure 1.2).

This image has been removed due to copyright issues.

Figure 1.2 Factors affecting the poor bioavailability for ocular dosage

1.5.2 Non-corneal Absorption

Apart from corneal route topically applied ocular drugs may be absorbed through non-corneal route. This route involves drug penetration across the bulbar conjunctiva and underlying sclera in to the uveal tract and vitreous humor. This route is important for hydrophilic and large molecules, such as insulin and p-aminoclonidine, which have poor corneal permeability.

1.6 DRAWBACKS OF TRADITIONAL OPHTHALMIC FORMULATIONS

1. They have poor bioavailability because of:
    a. Rapid precorneal elimination
    b. Conjunctival absorption
    c. Solution drainage by gravity
    d. Induced lacrimation
    e. Normal tear turnover
2. Frequent instillation of concentrated medication is required to achieve a therapeutic effect.
3. Systemic absorption of the drug and additives drained through nasolacrimal duct may result in undesirable side effects.
4. The amount of drug delivered during external application may vary. The drop size of ocular medication is not uniform and those delivered is generally not correct.
5. Presence of viscous vehicles can cause blurred vision.

1.7 CONJUNCTIVITIS

Conjunctivitis is an inflammation of the conjunctiva. It affects people of all ages. Acute conjunctivitis from various etiologies is characterized by common symptoms and signs including a red eye, discharge, eyelash matting or crusting, foreign body sensation, and tearing.

1.7.1 Common Causes of Conjunctivitis

Conjunctivitis is usually caused by infection or allergy. It is frequently referred to as "pink eye" and is the most common acute eye disorder seen by primary care pediatricians and family physicians. Typically, it is caused by a virus more often than bacteria. The cause of allergic conjunctivitis is an allergic reaction of the body's immune system to an allergen. Allergic conjunctivitis is common in people who have other signs of allergic disease such as hay fever, asthma and eczema (Bielory et al., 2007).

1.7.2 Allergic Conjunctivitis

Allergic conjunctivitis occurs very frequently. It is estimated to affect 20 percent of the population on an annual basis and approximately one-half of these people have a personal or family history of atopy. Allergic conjunctivitis may be divided into five major subcategories including 1) Seasonal allergic conjunctivitis, 2) Perennial allergic conjunctivitis, 3) Vernal keratoconjunctivitis, 4) Atopic keratoconjunctivitis and 5) Giant papillary conjunctivitis (Buckleyet al., 1998).

Seasonal (SAC) and perennial allergic conjunctivitis (PAC) combine to account for about two thirds of all allergic eye disease cases. The prevalence of SAC and PAC tends to be the same as hay fever or allergic rhinitis. Atopic keratoconjunctivitis is a bilateral, severe, allergic inflammation of the conjunctiva found in a subset of patients with atopic dermatitis. Atopic dermatitis occurs in 3% of the population and 15-40% of these will develop atopic keratoconjunctivitis. Vernal Keratoconjunctivitis is a bilateral, severe, vision threatening allergic inflammation of the conjunctiva (Weekeet al., 1987).

1.7.3 Treatment

Treatment consists of removal of any specific environmental triggers and a combination of supportive care including cool compresses and artificial tears for mild cases. The use of topical medications is reserved for more moderate cases and includes a combination of vasoconstrictors/antihistamines, mast cell stabilizers, non steroidal anti-inflammatory agents, and cyclosporine. Topical steroids may be used in severe cases. A trial of oral antihistamines is frequently utilized for moderate disease (Bielory L 2008).

1.8 NANOPARTICLES FOR OCULAR DRUG DELIVERY

Nanoparticles are defined as particles with a diameter of less than 1µm, comprising of various biodegradable or non-biodegradable polymers, lipids, phospholipids. Nanoparticles provide sustained release and prolonged therapeutic action, while retained in the cul-de-sac after topical administration and the entrapped drug to be released from the particles at an appropriate rate. Nanoparticles can be made of great variety of materials. Some of the most commonly used biomaterials include polyacrylates, polyalkylcyanoacrylates, polylactide (PLA), polylactide-polyglycolide (PLGA),polycaprolactones, dextran, albumin, gelatin, alginate, collagen, hyaluronic acid andchitosan (Diebold et al., 2010). Nanoparticles were considered to offer the possibility of amore facile delivery and transport across tissues. Alternatives to intravitreal or periocular injections, including scleral implants and devices, transdermal patches, and differention to phoretic devices including hydrogel reservoirs, have been explored with variable results. The underlying idea is to take advantage of the vitreous capacity for retaining and delivering molecules to tissues with which it is in direct contact and to use it as a biological reservoir once the nanoparticles are placed inside. There are promising studies reported in the recent literature on the use of intravitreally injected nanoparticles (Diebold et al., 2010).

1.8.1 Types of Nanoparticles (Torchilin, 2006)

1.8.1.1First Generation: Nanoparticles and Nanocapsules for Topical Ocular Delivery

Nanoparticles, primarily developed for intravenous administration, were first proposed for ophthalmic drug delivery in 1980. Different types of polymers including acrylic polymers and especially poly (alkyl cyanoacrylates) (PACA), polyesters, i.e., poly-ecaprolactone, and polysaccharides such as hyaluronic acid and chitosan have been reported for ocular drug delivery.

1.8.1.2 Second Generation Nanoparticles: Hydrophilic Polymer Coating Approach

The previously described nanoparticulate polymer-based carriers are shown to increase the intensity and contact time of drugs with the eye moreover, in some cases this improved contact led to an enhanced intraocular penetration of drugs. Taking this into account, a different approach has arisen based on the principle of providing to the nanocarrier, a polymer coating that favours its interaction with the ocular mucosa.

1.8.1.3 Third Generation: Surface Functionalized Carriers

In the particular case of the ocular drug delivery, the design of highly sophisticated drug delivery nano systems could benefit from the knowledge gained from the application of such systems to other trasmucosal routes of administration.

1.8.2 Advantages of Nanoparticles

Particle size and surface characteristics of nanoparticles can be easily manipulated to achieve both passive and active drug targeting after parenteral administration. Controlled release and particle degradation characteristics can be readily modulated by the choice of matrix constituents.

- Drug loading is relatively high and drugs can be incorporated into system without any chemical reaction which is an important factor for preserving the drug activity
- Sustained drug release and prolonged therapeutic activity
- Site-specific targeting -surface modification with ligands
- Protect the drug from chemical or enzymatic hydrolysis
- Efficient in crossing membrane barriers -blood retinal barrier
- Act as an inert carrier for ophthalmic drugs
- More stable than colloidal system

1.8.3 Preparation of Nanoparticles

The polymers are structured into nanometric size range by using appropriate methodologies which are enlisted below:

(i) Amphiphilic macromolecule cross-linking

    (a) Heat cross-linking

    (b) Chemical cross-linking

(ii) Polymerization based methods:

    (a) Polymerization of monomers *in situ*

    (b) Emulsion polymerization

    (c) Dispersion polymerization

    (d) Interfacial condensation polymerization

    (e) Interfacial complexation

(iii) Polymeric precipitation Methods

    (a) Solvent extraction / evaporation

(b) Nanoprecipitation

(c) Salting out

A number of different polymers have evaluated for the development of oral vaccines, included naturally polymers and synthetic polymers that include Sodium alginate, Chitosan, Polyactic acid (PLA), Polycaprolactone (PCL), Polylacide-co-glycolide (PLGA), Cyclodextrins.

1.9   OCULAR GELS

The most common way to improve drug retention on the corneal surface is undoubtedly by using polymers to increase solution viscosity. Hydrogels are polymers endowed with an ability to swell in water or aqueous solvents and induce a liquid–gel transition. Currently, two groups of hydrogels are distinguished, namely pre-formed gels, and *in situ* forming gels.

1.9.1 Pre-formed Gels

Preformed hydrogels can be defined as simple viscous solutions which do not undergo any modifications after administration. These typically utilize polymers such as polyvinyl alcohol (PVA), polyacrylamide, hydroxypropyl methylcellulose, hydroxypropyl cellulose, hydroxyethyl cellulose etc. The mechanisms of drug release involve a combination of diffusion from gel and erosion of gel surface.

1.9.2 *In situ* forming Gels

The use of preformed gels still has a number of lacunae which has limited their use in ophthalmic drug delivery. Administration of an accurate dose in the eye is one of the difficulties encountered with preformed gels owing to the variation of the amount of drug delivered during topical administration (Gutler et al.,, 1995). Due to resistance to eyelid motion, highly viscous solutions are often associated with discomfort and blurred vision. Thus *in situ* gel formulations are applied as solutions, sols, or suspensions which undergo gelation after instillation due to physic-chemical changes inherent to the eye. (Gurny*et al.,* 1993; Felt *etal.,* 1999)

1.9.2.1Thermo-reversible Sol to Gel Formulations

These formulations remain in the solution form at 20-25°C, however, upon instillation to eye, gelation occur due to increase in the temperature to 37°C. Different thermally setting polymers are available such as N-isopropyl acrylamide derivatives, acrylic acid copolymers etc. However specific requirements have restricted the use of such polymers.

Poloxamer are novel thermo reversible polymers that are widely used in sol-to-gel formulations. These give colorless and transparent gels. Another group of polymers widely used is cellulose derivatives such as methylcellulose, Hydroxyl propyl methyl cellulose (HPMC), Hydroxy ethyl cellulose (HEC). Methyl cellulose solutions transform into opaque gels between 40-50°C whereas HPMC shows phase transition at 75-90°C. Xyloglucan, a hemi cellulose derived from tamarind seed has also been used as thermo responsive polymer in sol to gel ocular delivery.

1.9.2.2 pH Sensitive Sol to Gel Formulations

These formulations remain in solution form at the relatively low pH of formulation and are transformed into gel form at pH 7.4 of tear fluid upon instillation. Cellulose acetate pseudo latexes and carbopol are the most widely used polymers in this category. Pseudo latexes are actually colloidal dispersion of polymers. Cellulose acetate phthalate latex (CAP-latex) forms free running solution at pH 4.2 and is converted into gel at pH 7.2.

1.9.2.3 Ionically Induced Sol to Gel Formulations

These formulations change to gel when come in contact with the ions present in the tear fluid. A very commonly used polymer to prepare these types of sol-to-gel formulation is Gelrite® which is a naturally occurring polymer (Carlfors et al., 1998).Another polymer showing ionically induced gelation property is alginic acid.

2.1 NANOPARTICLES

Chaiyasan et al., (2013) prepared mucoadhesive chitosan- dextran sulfate nanoparticles for sustained drug delivery to ocular surface. Rhodamine B, and nile red NR dye to determine the release pattern. Nanoparticles were synthesized by chitosan and dextran sulfate using poly electrolyte complexation method. The developed nanoparticulate system was able to overcome the short residence time of topical delivery through their sustained release and mucoadhesive character.

Gupta et al., (2013) developed a nanoparticles laden in situ gel for sustained ocular delivery. The authors used poly lactic co-glycolic acid for formulating nanoparticles employing nanoprecipitation method. The nanoparticles were loaded with sparfloxacin. The developed nanoparticulate system was dispersed into chitosan based *in situ* gelling system. From the release study it was concluded that the system was able to sustain the drug release and also enhance the precorneal residence time due to mucoadhesive nature of chitosan.

Kumar et al., (2012) worked on optimization and evaluation of short term tolerability of novel levofloxacin loaded PLGA Nanoparticles formulation. The nanoparticles were developed by using Emulsion-diffusion-evaporation method. The excipients used for nanoparticles preparation included poly(lactic-co-glycolic acid), Acetonitrile and dichloromethane. The developed nanoparticulate system had potential to produce sustain the release of levofloxacin.

Kaur et al., (2012) used carboxymethyl tamarind kernel polysaccharide for nanoparticles preparation. The carboxymethyl tamarind kernel powder was crosslinked with dioctyl sodium sulfo succinate using ionotropic gelation method. Tropicamide was loaded onto the carboxymethyl tamarind kernel polysaccharide based nanoparticles for ocular delivery. The formulated nanopaticles showed excellent ocular tolerability and mucoadhesive characters.

Aksungur et al., (2011) developed and characterized cyclosporine-A loaded nanoparticles for ocular delivery. The nanoparticles were prepared using either poly-lactide -co- glycolide (PLGA) or a mixture of PLGA with Eudragit RL, finally coated with Carbopol. The nanoparticulate system was developed using o/w emulsification solvent evaporation method followed by lyophilization. The cyclosporine loaded nanoparticulate system was able to sustain the drug release in the cul-de-sac for extended period of time and hence proved to be efficient delivery system for management of Keratoconjunctivitis sicca.

Nagarwal. et al., (2011) developed a modified PLA nano *in situ* gel as a potential ophthalmic drug delivery system for ocular delivery of 5-fluorouracil. The nanoparticles were formulated using nanoprecipitation method by employing poly(lactic acid) and PVA. The developed PLA nanoparticles loaded with 5- fluorouracil were dispersed in an *in situ* gelling base of sodium alginate. On *in vitro* and *in vivo* evaluation of the novel delivery system the MNS showed its potential for an effective targeting of the anterior ocular segment.

Rajendran et al., (2011) formulated acyclovir loaded chitosan nanoparticles for ocular delivery. The nanoparticles were prepared by ionotropic gelation method using chitosan as the matrix forming polymer and sodium tripolyphosphate as anionic crosslinker. The developed nanoparticles were to sustain the drug release and hence could decrease the administration frequency.

Das et al., (2011) designed a eudragit RS 100 nanoparticles for ocular delivery of Amphotericin B. Eudragit RS 100 nanoparticles were synthesized by nanoprecipitation, while the Solvent displacement process was used to entrap Amphotericin B in the nanosuspension. The developed nanosuspension had good retention property due to unique particle size and *in vitro* studies show attention for antifungal effect and minimal eye irritating effect.

Mahmoud et al., (2011) synthesized Chitosan/sulfobutyl-β-cyclodextrin nanoparticles for ocular delivery of econazole. Chitosan nanoparticles were synthesized using ionotropic gelation method using sulfobutylether-β-cyclodextrin (SBE-β-CD) as polyanionic crosslinker which could crosslink with cationic polymer chitosan. The developed formulation show zero order release kinetics, and also possessed mucoadhesive property that enabled the system to interact with ocular mucosa for extended period.

Gupta et al., (2010) developed sparfloxacin loaded PLGA nanoparticles. The nanoparticles were synthesized by nanoprecipitation method using sparfloxacin and PLGA, PVA. Formulated nanosuspension gave appropriate particle size, extended release with better tolerability and prolonged retention due to smaller particle size despite the anionic nature of PLGA polymer.

Mandal et al., (2009) developed and characterized chloramphenicol loaded biodegradable nanoparticle. The nanoparticles were synthesized using PLGA, PVA and ethyl acetate by solvent evaporation method. The system was able to prolong drug release as compared to free drug solution.

Yuan et al., (2008) prepared rapamycin loaded nanoparticles for immunesupresssion in corneal transplantation. The excipients used included chitosan, cholesterol 1-ethyl-3-(3-dimethylaminopropyl) carbodimide Poly lactic acid. The PLA based NPs were prepared by through nanoprecipitation method using cholesterol-modified chitosan as a stabilizer. Rapamycin loaded chitosan/PLA nanoparticles when used to treat corneal allograft, an excellent immunosuppressive effect was obsered along with better precorneal retention.

Papadimitriou et al., (2008) developed chitosan nanoparticles loaded with dorzolamide and pramipexol. The drug loaded nanoparticles were synthesized by ionotropic gelation method using chitosan and tripolyphosphate. The developed formulation showed sustained *in vitro* drug release and efficient mucoadhesive strength.

Motwani et al., (2008), developed chitosan-sodium alginate nanoparticles as submicroscopic reservoirs for ocular delivery of gatifloxacin. Chitosan–alginate polyionic complexes were formed through the modified coacervation via interactions between the carboxyl groups of alginate and the amine groups of chitosan. The drug release was more sustained in nanoparticles than conventional eye drops.

17

Banerjee et al., (2007) developed and compared ciprofloxacin hydrochloride loaded protein, lipid and chitosan nanoparticles for drug delivery. Polymers used included Bovine serum albumin, Glutaraldehyde, Stearic acid, Sodium taurocholate, Mannitol, Pentasodium TPP and Phosphatidyl choline. Desolvation based coacervation method was used for preparation of protein and gelatin nanoparticles, solid lipid nanoparticles were prepared by warm o/w microemulsion method while ionotropic gelation was used for formulating chitosan nanoparticles. The nanoaprticles were found to be promising formulation for prolong release of ciprofloxacin as compared to protein nanoparticles.

Agnihotri et al., (2007) developed chitosan nanoparticle for prolonged delivery of timolol maleate by desolvation technique using glutaraldehyde as crosslinking agent for polymeric chain of chitosan and sodium metabisulfite to stop the crosslinking. The nanoparticles showed prolonged delivery of timolol maleate, release was found to depend upon the extent of matrix crosslinking as well as molecular weight of CS. There was a continuous retardation in release with increase in crosslinking density.

Gan et al., (2007) developed chitosan nanoparticle as protein delivery carrier along with examination of fabrication condition for efficient drug loading and release. The model protein used was bovine serum albumin. Chitosan nanoparticle were fabricated by polyionic coacervation method while the protein loading was done both by incorporation and incubation. With the variation of chitosan and TPP, the release was modified due to the change in crosslinking density. On examination of TEM images, the release mechanism was follow desorption, diffusion and polymer erosion during different stages of release.

Huang et al., (2006) formulated a core shell type of nanoparticles composed of poly (n- butyl cyanoacrylate)-10-(2-octyl cyanoacrylate) for drug delivery. The core shell system was efficiently used for delivery of antibiotics Penicillin and streptomycin. The polymers used for developing the core shell structure included n-butyl cyanoacrylate 2-octyl cyanoacrylate Pluronic F127, DMSO. The nanoparticles of PBCA were prepared individually by emulsion polymerization technique. Poly (BCA-Co-OCA) feasible to encapsulate hydrophobic drug efficiently.

Vandervoort et al., (2004) prepared and evaluated drug loaded gelatin nanoparticles for topical ophthalmic use. For formulation of nanoparticles both gelatin type A and type B were used and applied as polymer, and pilocarpine hydrochloride and hydrocortisone were used as drugs. Desolvation technique was used for fabrication of drug loaded nanoparticles. Attempt was made to predict the release mechanism from gelatin nanoparticles. The r^2 values observed for the hydrocortisone loaded nanoparticles were close to 1, but not as close as the values found for pilocarpine HCl loaded nanoparticles. Hence assumption was made that the hydrocortisone release mechanism was anomalous, but close to zero order.

Pignatello et al., (2002) formulated acrylate nanoparticles for ophthalmic application. The flurbiprofen loaded nanoparticles were prepared by using eudragit RS100 and eudragit RL100 by 100 quasi-emulsion solvent diffusion technique. Nanoparticles were retained for a longer time.

Foucher et al., (2002) designed poly-ε-caprolactone nanospheres coated with bioadhesive hyaluronic acid for ocular delivery. The nanoparticulate system was developed by nanoprecipitation technique, and finally coated with hyaluronic acid coating was done to impart mucoadhesive character to the delivery system. The system was used to prolong the precorneal residence time due to surface positive charge provided by the hyaluronic acid.

Guan et al., (2001) worked on optimization of preparation conditions for levofloxacin loaded chitosan nanoparticles. The nanoparticles were synthesized by ionotropic gelation method in which a orthogonal experiment was applied by varying the level and mass ratio of chitosan and TPP. The developed nanoparticles were able to sustain the drug release for three days.

De Campos et al., (2001) developed chitosan nanoparticles for the improvement of the drug delivery to ocular surface. The nanoparticles were synthesized using ionic gelation method employing sodium tripolyphosphate as anionic crosslinker. The developed system was able to provide a sustained drug delivery to external ocular tissue, specifically thus maintaining a long term drug level on ocular surface.

Desai et al., (2000) prepared biodegradable polyisobutylcyano-acrylate nanocapsule for ocular delivery of pilocarpine. Pilocarpine loaded polyisobutylcyano-acrylate nanoparticles were prepared by interfacial polymerization technique. The developed system was able to increase the corneal contact time between pilocarpine and ocular absorbing tissue thereby improving bioavailability of drug.

Fresta et al., (2000) assessed ocular tolerability and *in vivo* bioavailability of polymeric nanospheres encapsulating acyclovir. Polymer were used for formulating nanoparticles included poly(ethylene glycol) ethyl-2-cyanoacrylate, Pluronic F68, PEG 6000, HP-β-cyclodextrin, and the nanoparticles were prepared by micellar polymerization. The poly ethyl cyanoacrylate nanospheres were coated with polyethylene glycol and were able to increase acyclovir ocular bioavailability compared with the raw drug, which may be due to better interaction with corneal epithelium.

Murakami et al., (1997) evaluated the influence of degree of hydrolyzation and polymerization on the preparation and properties of PLGA nanoparticles. The PLGA nanoparticles were prepared by spontaneous emulsion solvent diffusion method. Twelve grades of PVA were used in the formulation of nanoparticulate system. Physical properties of PLGA nanoparticles were determined by the grade of PVA used with hydrolyzation affecting most significantly the characteristics of nanoparticles.

Cavattaro et al., (1994) developed polyethyl cyanoacrylate nanoparticles for entrapment of β-lactam antibiotics. The β-lactam antibiotics used in the system were cefaclor monohydrate and cefsulodin. The nanoparticles were prepared by micellar polymerization utilizing ethyl 2-cyanoacrylate and polyethylene poly propylene as the matrix forming polymer. Prepared nanoparticles showed prolong release.

Heussler et al., (1990) determined the antiglaucomatous activity of (betaxolol chlorhydrate) sorbed into different isobutyl cyanoacrylate nanoparticle. The nanoparticles were prepared via desolvation method using isobutyl cyanoacrylate, dextran 70000, dextran sulfate N-acetyl glucosamine. The system tends to show long residence time of the particles in the cul-de-sac and hence increased the drug bioavailability.

2.2 OCULAR *IN SITU* GELS

Rozier et al., (1989) were prepared novel ion activated *in situ* gelling using Gelrite as a polymer for ophthalmic vehicles and a 0.6 % Gelrite vehicle has been compared to an equiviscous solution of hydroxy ethyl cellulose using Timolol Maleate as a drug probe. They were observed that *in vivo*; the formation of the gel prolonged precorneal residence time and increased ocular bioavailability of timolol.

Lindell et al., (1993) showed *in vitro* release of Timolol Maleate from an *in situ* gelling polymer, cellulose ether [ethyl (hydroxy ethyl) cellulose] system. They were observed that the release of Timolol Maleate was about equal for system with 1-2 % w/w EHEC, implying that the release was controlled by a low convection in the gels and not by any drug-polymer interaction.

Kumar et al (1994) prepared a *in situ* forming gels by a combination of Carbopol and Methylcellulose and carried out the rheological characterization of such system at two different pH (4 and 7) and temperatures (25° and 37°C). They found that an increase in concentration of either Carbopol or Methylcellulose resulted in an increase in viscosity and shear stress among the compositions. A solution containing 1.5 % Methylcellulose, 0.3 % Carbopol was found to have low viscosity and formed a strong gel under simulated physiological conditions.

Kumar et al., (1995) studied modification of *in situ* gelling behavior of Carbopol solutions by HPMC. They found that in combination, both HPMC and

22

Carbopol form low viscosity liquid at pH 4 and transform into stiff gels with plastic rheological behavior and comparable viscosities upon increasing the pH up to 7.4. HPMC-PAA gels show slow *in vitro* release of incorporated Timolol Maleate.

Cohen S et al., (1997) developed a novel *in situ* gel forming ophthalmic drug delivery system from Alginate undergoing gelation in the eye. They demonstrated that an aqueous solution of sodium alginate could gel in the eye, without the addition of external calcium ions or other bivalent/polyvalent cations. Alginate with guluronic acid contents of more than 65 %, such as Manugel DMB, instantaneously formed gels upon their addition to simulated lachrymal fluid, while those having low guluronic acid contents, such as Ketton LV, formed weak gels at a relatively slow rate and hence it was indicated that the *in situ* gelling Alginate system, based on polymers with high guluronic acid contents, was an excellent drug carrier for the prolonged delivery of Pilocarpine.

Dimitrova et al., (2000) developed a model of aqueous ophthalmic solution of Indomethacin on the basis of Pluronic F68 and Pluronic F127. They showed that both Pluronics acted very similarly and were effective as solubilizers, created an appropriate viscosity, and formed reversible gels at higher temperature, ensured the chemical stability of indomethacin and prolonged *in vitro* drug diffusion, and showed high physiological tolerance in rabbit eyes.

Sechoy et al., (2000) developed a new long acting ophthalmic formulation of Carteolol containing alginic acid. They observed that the alginic acid vehicle is an excellent drug carrier, well tolerated, and could be used for the development of a long-acting ophthalmic formulation of Carteolol. *In vitro* studies indicated that Carteolol was released slowly from Alginic acid formulation, suggesting an ionic interaction.

Hong-Ru Lin, et al (2000) developed Carbopol/Pluronic phase change solution for ophthalmic drug delivery. The results demonstrated that the Carbopol/Pluronic mixture could be used as an *in situ* gelling vehicle to enhance the ocular bioavailability.

Srividya et al., (2001) prepared sustained ophthalmic delivery of ofloxacin from a pH triggered *in situ* gelling system using Polyacrylic acid (Carbopol 940), as the gelling agent in combination with HPMC E50LV. They observed that the developed formulation was therapeutically efficacious, stable, non-irritating and provided sustained release of the drug over an 8 h period.

Miyazaki et al., (2001) prepared *in situ* gelling Xyloglucan formulations for sustained release ocular delivery of Pilocarpine HCL. They found that the degree of enhancement of mitotic response following sustained release of Pilocarpine from 1.5 % w/w Xyloglucan gel was similar to that from a 25 % w/w Pluronic F127 gel.

El-Kamel et al., (2000) demonstrated *in vitro/in vivo* evaluation of Pluronic F127-based ocular delivery system for timolol maleate. They observed that the slowest drug release was obtained from 15% Pluronic F127 formulation containing 3% methyl cellulose. *In vivo* study showed that the ocular bioavailability of Timolol Maleate, increased by 2.5 and 2.4 fold for 25% Pluronic F127 gel formulation and 15% Pluronic F127 containing 3% methyl cellulose respectively, compared with 0.5% timolol maleate aqueous solution.

Charoo et al., (2002) prepared *in situ* forming ophthalmic gels of Ciprofloxacin HCl for the treatment of bacterial conjunctivitis, using HPMC K15 M and Carbopol 934. They demonstrated that the sol-to-gel system exhibited a zero-order drug release pattern over 24 h in *in vitro* release studies.

Sultana et al., (2006) evaluated carbopol-methyl cellulose based sustained release ocular delivery system for pefloxacin mesylate using rabbit eye model. It was found that the optimum concentration of carbopol solution for *in situ* gel forming delivery system was 0.3% w/w and that for methyl cellulose solution was 1.5% w/w. The mixture of solutions showed a significant enhancement in gel strength in the physiological condition. Both *in vitro* and *in vivo*, indicated the carbopol and methyl cellulose solutions alone and mixture can be used as an *in situ* gelling vehicle to enhance the ocular bioavailability of Pefloxacin Mesylate.

Liu et al., (2006) studied an Alginate/ HPMC based *in situ* gelling ophthalmic delivery system for Gatifloxacin. They observed that the Alginate/HPMC solution retained the drug better than the Alginate or HPMC E50LV solutions alone and mixture can be used as *in situ* gelling vehicle to enhance ocular bioavailability and patient compliance.

Rao et al., (2006) developed a phase transition system of timolol maleate for glaucoma treatment to prolonged acting ocular drug delivery in glaucoma therapy, using carbopol 971P with added viscolizers like HEC, HPMC and MC. They observed that the gradual decrease in intraocular pressure and maintaining the same for prolonged periods and it was mainly due to viscosity of the formulation, which helps in sustained release of timolol maleate.

Qi et al., (2007) developed a Polaxomer analogs/Carbopol based *in situ* gelling and mucoadhesive ophthalmic delivery system for Puerarin. They observed that the incorporation of Carbopol 1342P NF not only did not affect the pseudoplastic behavior with hysteresis of the Polaxomer analogs solutions and leaded to a higher shear stress at each shear rate, but also enhanced the mucoadhesive force significantly. It was indicated that the combined solution had better ability to retain drug than Polaxomer analogs or Carbopol alone.

Wu et al, (2007) prepared and evaluated a Carbopol 980 NF/HPMC E4M based *in situ* gelling ophthalmic system for Puerarin. They observed that when these two vehicles were combined, an *in situ* gel with the appropriate gel strength and gelling capacity under physiological conditions. This combined solution flowed freely under non-physiological condition and showed the character of pseudoplastic fluid under both conditions. The combined polymer systems performed better in retaining Puerarin than Puerarin eye drops.

Mitan et al., (2000) prepared a pH induced *in situ* gel forming ophthalmic drug delivery system for Tropicamide. They used Polyacrylic acid 940 as the gelling agent in combination with HPMC K15M as a viscosity-enhancing agent. They developed formulation provided sustained release of drug at the site of action over 8 h. The selected formulation was tested in albino rabbits (male) using the Draize test protocol with crossover studies and found to be non-irritant to the rabbit eye.

Thilekkumak et al., (2005) prepared pH induced *in situ* gelling system of indomethacin for sustained ocular delivery. They observed that the Carbopol solution which are acidic and less viscous, transformed into stiff gels upon increase in pH of tear fluid of the eye, as the gelling agents and its combination with HPMC K15M. The obtained therapeutic efficacy and sustained release of Indomethacin over 8 h period, which made them an excellent candidate for *in situ* gelling ocular delivery system.

Kulkarni et al. (2007) prepared the ophthalmic *in situ* gelling formulation of Flubiprofen Sodium using gellan gum. The formulation in gel form showed almost complete release of drug. The formulation when subjected to accelerated stability studies showed good physical and chemical stability and the *in vivo* studies of the formulation in albino rabbits confirmed its *in situ* gelling ability as well as non-irritating, non toxic nature.

One of the main and still-remaining problems in ophthalmic drug delivery is the rapid elimination of conventional liquid eye-drops. Many factors lead to a high rate of lacrimal drainage. Rapid tear turnover resulting precorneal drug loss, induction of tear flow due to irritation caused by eye drops, relatively large volume of the administered eye drops, are few factors responsible for drainage and these still remain unsolved. Due to the resulting elimination rate, the precorneal half-life of drugs is considered to be between about 1-3 min. As a consequence, only a very small amount (1-3% of the total administered dose) dosage actually penetrates through the cornea and reaches intraocular tissues.

Conjunctivitis is one of the common ocular disorder, characterized by inflammation of eye, which results in redness and irritation of eye. The existing therapy with conventional eye drops is fairly primitive and inefficient due to nasolachrymal drainage, which results in reduced corneal residence time of the drug.

To overcome this undesirable aspect of eye drops, in the present work, on attempt has been made to develop controlled release *in situ* gel incorporating nanoparticles, using natural and semi synthetic polymers, for the treatment of conjunctivitis.

Azelastine HCl and Cromolyn sodium are the drugs of choice in management of allergic conjunctivitis. It is envisaged to develop ocular *in situ* gels incorporating nanoparticles of both anti allergic agents which provides dual advantages of nanoparticle system and the gel. Nanoparticles are aimed at improving the precorneal residence time of dosage form at ocular surface, which can improve absorption. *In situ* gel forming systems are viscous liquids that undergo phase transition to form a viscoelastic gel upon exposure to physiological conditions (pH or temperature). They deliver the drug in accurate and reproducible quantities, are convenient to administer and promote precorneal retention. They capable of delivering the drug in a sustained manner, thus avoiding frequent instillation and prevent local and systemic toxic effects. Thus *in situ* gel forming system incorporating nanoparticles may by increase corneal residence as well as conjunctival penetration.

REFERENCES

1. Agnihotri, S.M. and Vavia, P.R. Diclofenac-loaded biopolymeric nanosuspensions for ophthalmic applications. Nanomed Nanotech Biol Med, 5, (1) (2009) 90-95.

2. Ahmed, I. and Patton, T.F.. Importance of the non-corneal absorption route in topical ophthalmic drug delivery. Invest. Ophthalmol. Vis. Sci, 26 (4) (1985) 584–587.

3. Aksungur, P., Demirbile, M., Denkbas, E.B., Vandervoort, J., Ludwig, A. and Unlu, N. Development and characterization of cyclosporine A loaded nanoparticles for ocular drug delivery: cellular toxicity, uptake and kinetic studies. J. Controlled Release. 151 (3) (2011) 286-94.

4. Ali, H.S., York, P., Ali, A.M. and Blagden N. Hydrocortisone nanosuspension for ophthalmic delivery: a comparative study between microfluidic nanopercipitation and wet milling. J. Controlled Release. 49 (2) (2011)175-81.

5. Avis KE, Lieberman HA, Lachman L. "Development of ophthalmic formulations". Pharmaceutical dosage forms: Parenteral medications. 2nd ed. New York: Marcel Dekker Inc.; (1993) 542-57.

6. BanarJ.ee R., J.ain D., 'Comparison of Ciprofloxacin Hydrochloride-Loaded Protein, Lipid, and Chitosan Nanoparticles for Drug Delivery', J.

Biomed. Mater. Res. Part B: Applied Biomat. (2007) 105-112.

7. Bielory L, Friedlaender MH. Allergic conjunctivitis. Immunol Allergy Clin North Am 28 (1) (2008) 43–58.

8. Bielory L, Katelaris CH, Lightman S. Treating the ocular component of allergic rhinoconJ.unctivitis and related eye disorders. Med Gen Med. 9 (3) (2007) 35-107.

9. Bourlais CL, Acar L, Zia H, Sado PA, Needhan S, Leverge R. Ophthalmic drug delivery systems – Recent Advances. Prog Retin Eye Res. 17 (1) (1998) 33-58.

10. Bruck SD. Controlled drug delivery. BocaRaton, Florida, : CRC Press; 1983.

11. Buckley RJ. "Allergic eye disease—a clinical challenge". Clin. Exp. Allergy 28 (6) (1998) 39–43.

12. Carlfors, J., Edsman., K., Petersson, R. And J.ornving, K., 1998. Rheological evaluation of gelrite in situ gels for ophthalmic use. Eur J. Pharm Sci , 6 (2) (1998) 113-119.

13. Cavallaro G., Fresta M., Giammona G., Pulgisi G. and Villari D. 'Entrapment of β-1actams antibiotics in polyethylcyanoacrylate nanoparticles: Studies on the possible in vivo application of this colloidal delivery system', Int. J. Pharm., 111, (1994) 31-41.

14. Charoo NA, Kohil K, Ali A. Preparation of In situ forming ophthalmic

gels of ciprofloxacin HCL for the treatment of conjunctivitis: In-vitro and In-vivo studies., J. Pharm. Sci., 92 (2) (2002) 407-13.

15.Chein, Y.W., Novel Drug Delivery System, Marcel Dekker, New York, 50 (1992) 269-289.

16.Cohen S, Lobel E, Trevgoda A, Peled Y. A Novel In situ forming ophthalmic drug delivery system from alginates undergoing gellation in the eye. J. of Controlled Release 44 (2-3) (1997) 201-8.

17.Coquelet C, Lakhchaf N, Persin M, Rao LS, Sarrazin J. Association between benzalkonium chloride and poly (Acrylic Acid) gel study by microfiltration and membrane dialysis., J. of Membr. Sci., 120 (2) (1996) 287-93.

18.Das S. and Suresh P.K. Nanosuspension: a new vehicle for the improvement of the delivery of drugs to the ocular surface. Application to amphotericin B, Nanomed. Nanotech. Bio. Med. 7 (2011) 242-247, doi:10.1016/J.nano.2010.07.003

19.De Campos A.M., Sanchez A. and Alonso M. J. 'Chitosan nanoparticles: a new vehicle for the improvement of the delivery of drugs to the ocular surface. Application to cyclosporin A', Int. J. Pharm., 224(2001) 159-168.

20.Desai S. D. and Blanchard J. 'Pluronic ®F127- based ocular delivery system containing biodegradable polyisobutylcyanoacrylate nanocapsule of pilocarpine', Drug Del., 7 (2000) 201–207.

21. Desai, S.D. and Blanchard, J., In vitro evaluation of Pluronic F-127 based controlled release ophthalmic delivery systems for pilocarpine., J. Pharm. Sci. 87 (1998) 226-230.

22. Diebold Y. and Calonge M. Application of nanoparticles in ophthalmology. Progress in Retinal and Eye Research, 29 (2010) 596-609.

23. Dimitrova E, Bogdanova SV, Mitcheva M, Tanev I, Minkov E. Development of model aqueous ophthalmic solution of indomethacin. Drug Development and Industrial Pharmacy 26 (12) (2000) 297-301.

24. Ding S. Recent Developments in ophthalmic drug delivery. Pharmaceutical sciences and technology Today 1(8) (1998) 328-35.

25. Edsman K, Carfors J., HarJ.u K. Rheological evaluation and ocular contact time of some carbomer gels for ophthalmic use. Int. J. Pharm., 137 (1996) 233-41.

26. Felt, O., Baeyens, V., Zignani, M., Buri, P. and Gurny, R. Mucosal drug delivery-ocular. Encyclopedia of controlled drug delivery 2, University of Geneva, Geneva, Switzerland, (1999) 605–622.

27. Fitzgerald, P., Wilson, C. G. Polymeric systems for ophthalmic drug delivery. In: Polymeric Biomaterials (S. Dimitriu, ed.) Marcel Dekker, New York. (1994) 373-398.

28. Foucher B, Grefa P., Russoa J., Guechotb J., Bochota A., (2002), 'Design of poly- β- Caprolactone nanospheres coated with bioadhesive hyaluronic acid for ocular delivery', J. Controlled Release, 83 (2002) 365–375.

29. Fresta M., Fontana G., Bucolo C., Cavalloro G., Giammona G. and Puglisi G. 'Ocular tolerability and in vivo bioavailability of poly ethylene glycol coated polyethyl-2-cyanoacrylate nanospheres encapsulated Acyclovir', J. Pharm. Sci. 90 (2001) 288-297.

30. Fulcher EM, Soto CD, Fulcher RM. "Medications for disorders of the eye and ear". In; pharmacology: Principles and applications. Philadelphia PA: Saunders; (2003)461-2.

31. Furrer, P., Plazonnet B., Mayer J.M., Gurny, R. Application of In vivo confocal microscopy to the obJ.ective evaluation of ocular irritation induced by surfactants. Int. J. Pharm., 207 (2000) 89-98.

32. Gan Q., Wang T. 'Chitosan nanoparticle as protein delivery carrier— Systematic examination of fabrication conditions for efficient loading and release', Colloids and surfaces B: bioInt.faces 59 (2007) 24-34.

33. Gaudana R., J.wala., Sai H., Boddu S. and Mitra A.K., 2009. Recent perspectives in ocular delivery. Pharmaceut Res. 26 (5) (2009) 1197-1216.

34. Gavini, E., Chetoni, P., Cossu, M., Alvarez, M.G., Saettone, M.F. and Giunchedi, P. PLGA microspheres for the ocular delivery of a peptide

drug, vancomycin using emulsification/spray-drying as the preparation method: in vitro/in vivo studies. Eur. J. Pharm. Biopharm, 57, (2004) 207–212.

35.Guana J., Chenga P., Huanga S. J., Wua J. M., Lia Z. H., Youa X. D., Haoa L M., Guoa Y., Lia R.X., Zhang H. ' Optimized preparation of levofloxacin-loaded chitosan nanoparticles by ionotropic gelation', Physics Procedia. 22, (2011) 163-169.

36.Gupta H., Aqil M., Khar R. K., Ali A., Bhatnagar A., Mittal G. 'Nanoparticles laden in situ gel for sustained ocular drug delivery', J. Pharm. Bioallied. Sci. 5 (2) (2013) 162-165.

37.Gupta, H., Aquil, M., Khar, R.K., Ali, A., Bhatnagar, A. and Mittal, G. Sparfloxacin- loaded PLGA nanoparticles for sustained ocular delivery. Nanomed. Nanotech. Bio. Med. 6 (2010) 324-333.

38.Gutler, F. and Gurny, R. Patent literature review of ophthalmic inserts. Drug Dev. Ind. Pharm., 21, (1) (1995)1-18.

39.Heussler, L.M., Maincent, P., Hoffman, M., Spittler, J. and Couvreur, P. Antiglaucomatous activity of betaxolol chlorhydrate sorbed different isobutylcyanoacrylate nanoparticles preparations., Int. J. Pharm., 58, (2) (1990) 115-122.

40.Huang C. and Lee Y. 'Core-shell type of nanoparticles composed of poly[(n-butyl cyanoacrylate)-co-(2-octyl cyanoacrylate)]copolymers for drug delivery application: Synthesis, characterization and in vitro degradation', Int. J. Pharm., 325 (2006) 132–139.

41. Kaur, H., AhuJ.a, M., Kumar, S. and Dilbaghi, N., 2012.Carboxymethyl tamarind kernel polysaccharide nanoparticles for ophthalmic drug delivery. Int. J. of Biol. Macromol., 50 (2012) 833-839.

42. Kulkarni MC, Damle AV. Development of ophthalmic in-situ gelling formulation of flurbiprofen sodium using gellan gum. Indian Drugs. 44 (5) (2007) 373-7.

43. Kumar G., Sharma S., Shafiq N. and Khuller G.K. 'Optimization, in vitro-in vivo evaluation, and short term tolerability of novel levofloxacin-loaded PLGA Nanoparticle formulation', J. Pharm. Sci., 101 (2012) 2165–2176.

44. Kumar S, Haglund BO, Himmelstein KJ. In-situ forming gels for ophthalmic drug delivery, J Ocul Pharmacol Ther. 10 (1) (1994):47-56.

45. Kumar S, Himmelstein KJ. Modification of in-situ gelling behavior of carbopol solutions by HPMC. J. Pharm. Sci., 84 (3) (1995) 344-8.

46. Lin H, Sung KC. Carbopol / pluronic phase change solution for ophthalmic drug delivery. J. of Controlled Release 69 (3) (2000) 379-88.

47. Lindell K. and Engstrom S., In Vitro Release of Timolol from An In Situ Gelling Polymer System, Int. J. Pharm 95(1-3) (1993) 219-28.

48. Liu Z, Li Z, Nie S, Liu H. Ding P and Pan W., Study of an alginate /

HPMC based In-situ gelling ophthalmic delivery system for gatifloxacin. Int. J. Pharm. 315(1-2) (2006)12-7.

49.Mahmoud A.A., Feky G.S., Kamel R. and Awad G.E.A. 'Chitosan/sulfobutylether -β-cyclodextrin nanoparticles as a potential approach for ocular delivery', Int. J. Pharm. (2011).

50.Mandal B., Halder K., Bey S.K., Bhoumik M., Debuath M.C. and Ghosh L.K. (2009) 'Development and physical characterization of chloramphenicol loaded biodegradable Nanoparticles for prolonged release', Mol. Vision. 64, (2009) 445-449.

51.Meqi, S.A., Deshpande, S.G. Controlled and novel drug delivery, CBS Publishers, New Delhi. (2002) 82-84.

52.Mitan R.G., Dharmesh M. M., Jolly R. P., In situ gel system for ocular drug delivery: A review. Drug Delivery Rev. 7 (3) (2007) 30-37.

53.Mitan RG, J.olly RP, Megha B, Dharmesh M.M. A pH triggered In-situ gel forming ophthalmic drug delivery system for tropicamide. Drug Delivery Technology. 7(5) (2007) 44-9.

54.Miyazaki S, Suzuki S, Kawasaki N, Endo K, Takahasi A, Attwood D. In-situ gelling xyloglucan formulation for sustained release ocular delivery of pilocarpine HCL. Int. J. Pharm. 229(1-2) (2007) 29-36.

55.Motwani S.K., Chopra S., Talegaonkar S., Kohli K., Ahmad F. J. and Khar R. K. 'Chitosan–sodium alginate nanoparticles as submicroscopic reservoirs for ocular delivery: Formulation, optimization and in vitro characterisation', Eur. J. Pharm. Biopharm, 68, (2007) 513–525.

56. Murakami H., Kawashima Y., Niwa T., Hino T., Takeuchi H. and Kobayashi. 'Influence Of degree of hydrolyzation and polymerization poly(vinylalcohol) on the preparation and properties of poly(DL-lactide-co-glycolide) nanoparticle', Int. J. Pharm. 149 (1097) 43-49.

57. Nagarwal R. C., Shri Kant, Singh P.N., Maiti P. and Pandit J.K. 'Polymeric nanoparticulate system: A potential approach for ocular drug delivery', J. Controlled Release 136 (2009) 2–13.

58. Nanjawade, B. K., Manvi,. F. V. and ManJ.appa, A. S. In situ-forming hydrogels for sustained ophthalmic drug delivery. J. of Controlled Release, 122, (2007) 119–134.

59. Ono, S. J., Abelson M.B. "Allergic conJ.unctivitis: update on pathophysiology and prospects for future treatment". J. Allergy Clin. Immunol. 115 (1) (2005) 118–22.

60. Papadimitriou S., Bikiaris D., Avgoustakis K., karavas E. and Georgarakis M. 'Chitosan nanoparticles loaded with dorzolamide and pramipexole' Carbo. Polym. 1 (4) (2008) 44-54.

61. Phate RP. "The eye and vision". In; anatomy, physiology and health education. 2nd ed. Nasik: career publication; (2003) 248

62. Pignatello R., Bucolo C., Ferrara P., Maltese A., Puleo A. and Pugisi G.

(2002) 'Eudragit RS 100 nanosuspension for the ophthalmic controlled delivery of Ibuprofen', Eur. J. Pharm. Biopharm., 16(1-2) (2002) 53-61.

63.Pignatello R., Bucolo C., Spedalieri G., Maltese A. and Puglisi G. (2002) 'Flurbiprofen- Loaded acrylate polymer nanopsuspension for ophthalmic application', Biomaterials, 23 (15) (2002) 3247-3255.

64.Qi H., Chen W, Huang C, Li L, Chen C, Li W. Development of a poloxamer analogs / carbopol based In-situ gelling and mucoadhesive ophthalmic delivery system for puerarin. Int. J. Phar (337) (2007)178-87.

65.Rajendran N. N., NatraJ.an R., Kumar R. S. and SelvaraJ. S. 'Acyclovir loaded chitosan nanoparticles for ocular delivery', Asian. J. Pharm. 4 (4) (2000) 220-226

66.Rao KP, Bushetti SS. Phase transition systems of timolol maleate for glaucoma treatment: prolonged acting ocular drug delivery in glaucoma therapy. Indian Drugs. 43(11) (2006) 909-13.

67.Chaiyasan W., Srinivas S P., Tiyaboonchai W., 'Mucoadhesive chitosan-dextran sulfate nanoparticles for sustained drug delivery to the ocular surface', J. Ocul. Pharmacol. Ther. 29, (2) (2012) 200-7.

68.Roizer A, Manzuel C,Grove J., Planzonnet B. Gelrite: A novel, ion-activated, in- Situ gelling polymer for ophthalmic vehicles effect on bioavailability of timolol. Int. J. Pharm. 1989; 57 (2) (1989) 62-80.

69.Sechoy O, Tissie G, Sebastian C, Maurin F, Driat J., Trinquand C. A New long acting ophthalmic formulation of carteolol containing alginic acid. Int. J. Pharm., 207 (2000) 109-116.

70. Srividya B, Cardoza RM, Amin PD. Sustained ophthalmic delivery of ofloxacin from a pH triggered in-situ gelling system. J. of Controlled Release. 73(2-3) (2001) 205-11.

71. Sultana Y, Aquil M, Ali A, Zafar S. Evaluation of carbopol-methyl cellulose based sustained release ocular delivery for pefloxacin desylate using rabbit eye model. Pharmaceutical Development Technologies 11(3) (2006) 313-9.

72. Thilekkumar M., Bharathi D., Balasubhramaniam J., Kant S. and Pandit J. K., pH-induced In situ gelling systems of indomethacin for sustained ocular delivery, Int. J. Pharm. Sci., 67(3) (2005) 327-33.

73. Tortora GJ., Grabowski SR, editors. Principles of anatomy and physiology. 10th ed. New York: John Wiley and Sons, Inc; 2003.

74. Unlu N, Ludwig A, Van OM, Hincal AA. Formulation of carbopol 940 ophthalmic vehicles, and In-vitro evaluation of the influence of simulated lacrimal fluid on their physico-chemical properties. Pharmazie. 46 (11) (1991) 784-8.

75. Vandervoort, J. and Ludwig, A. 'Preparation and evaluation of drug-loaded gelatin nanoparticles for topical ophthalmic use' Eur. J. Pharm. Biopharm. 57 (2) (2004) 251-61.

76. Wagh A, Grant A, editors. Ross and Wilson Anatomy and Physiology in Health and Illness. 9th ed. London: Churchill Livingstone; 2001.

77. Weeke ER. Epidemiology of hay fever and perennial allergic rhinitis. Monogr Allergy. 21(1987) 1–20.

78. Wu C, Qi H, Chen W, Hung C, Su C, Li W. Preparation and evaluation of a carbopol / HPMC based In-situ gelling ophthalmic system for puerarin. Yakugaku Zasshi 127(1) (2007) 183-91.

79. Yuan X. B., Yuan Y. B., J.iang W., Liu J., Tian E. and Shun H. (2008) 'preparation of rapamycin-loaded chitosan /PLA nanoparticle for immune-suppression in corneal transplantation', Int. J. Pharm. 349 (2008) 241-248.

YOUR KNOWLEDGE HAS VALUE

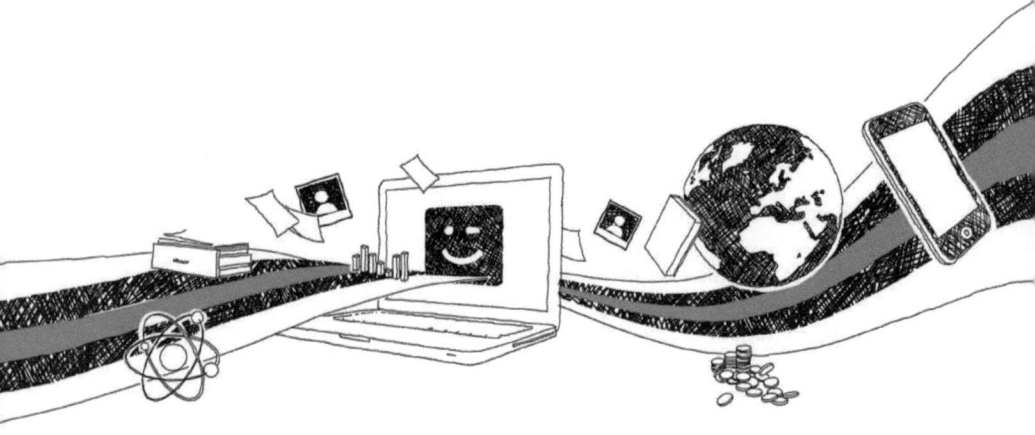

- We will publish your bachelor's and
  master's thesis, essays and papers

- Your own eBook and book -
  sold worldwide in all relevant shops

- Earn money with each sale

Upload your text at www.GRIN.com
and publish for free

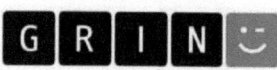